ANGER MANAGEMENT FOR PARENTS

A Guide for Parents to Manage Anger and Stay Calm

MELISSA J. POWELL

TABLE OF CONTENT

INTRODUCTION

Once upon a time in the town of Harmonyville, there were parents facing a common challenge – managing their anger. Imagine a day when Mr. and Mrs. Johnson found themselves feeling frustrated and upset. Instead of yelling or getting mad, they decided to learn the magical art of anger management. Join them on a journey to discover simple tips and tricks that helped them create a happier home for their family. This story is here to share those secrets and help parents turn angry moments into moments of calm and understanding. So, let's embark on this adventure together!

CHAPTER 1

Understanding Anger

Understanding anger is a crucial aspect of emotional intelligence and personal growth. Anger, often considered a negative emotion, is a natural and universal human experience. It can manifest in various intensities, from mild irritation to intense rage, and can be triggered by internal or external factors.

At its core, anger is an emotional response to a perceived threat or injustice. Understanding the roots of anger involves delving into its psychological, physiological, and evolutionary aspects. Psychologically, anger can be a defense mechanism, a way for individuals to assert boundaries and protect themselves. Physiologically, the body responds to anger by releasing stress hormones, preparing for a "fight or flight" response. Evolutionarily, anger may have served as a survival mechanism, aiding in confrontations with threats.

One important aspect of understanding anger is recognizing its triggers. These triggers can be diverse, ranging from personal frustrations to external stressors. Identifying these triggers empowers individuals to address the root causes of their anger and implement effective coping mechanisms. For example, a parent dealing with work stress may unintentionally bring that frustration home, leading to anger in family situations. By acknowledging the source of anger, one can work towards finding healthier ways to cope with stress and prevent it from impacting relationships.

Moreover, it's essential to distinguish between healthy and unhealthy expressions of anger. Healthy anger involves acknowledging and expressing the emotion in a constructive manner. This may include calmly discussing concerns, setting boundaries, or seeking support. Unhealthy anger, on the other hand, involves aggressive or destructive behavior that can harm oneself or others. Understanding this distinction is vital for cultivating emotional intelligence and fostering positive relationships.

Another crucial aspect of understanding anger is the role of communication. Effective communication is a powerful tool for managing anger. Often, anger arises from miscommunication or unmet expectations. Learning to express feelings and needs assertively, while also actively listening to others, can prevent misunderstandings that lead to anger. In family settings, open and honest communication is especially important to maintain harmonious relationships.

In addition, introspection plays a key role in understanding and managing anger. Reflecting on one's emotional responses, triggers, and patterns of behavior provides valuable insights. Journaling or seeking the guidance of a therapist can facilitate this self-exploration process. By understanding the underlying causes of anger, individuals can develop self-awareness and make conscious choices in how they respond to challenging situations.

Furthermore, the impact of childhood experiences on anger management cannot be overlooked. Early life experiences, such as family dynamics and upbringing, significantly influence how individuals express and cope with anger. Those raised in environments where anger was handled constructively may develop healthier anger management skills, while others may struggle if exposed to aggressive or suppressive approaches. Acknowledging and addressing these early influences is an integral part of understanding and transforming one's relationship with anger.

Cognitive restructuring is a powerful technique in understanding and managing anger. This involves challenging and changing negative thought patterns that contribute to anger. For example, someone prone to perfectionism may become excessively angry when things don't go as planned. By reevaluating these unrealistic expectations and adopting a more flexible mindset, individuals can reduce the likelihood of anger arising in such situations.

Moreover, empathy plays a pivotal role in understanding anger, both in oneself and others. Empathizing with the perspectives and emotions of those around us fosters compassion and defuses potential conflicts. Parents, for instance, can benefit greatly from empathizing with their children's feelings, helping create an environment where open communication and understanding prevail.

Lastly, developing effective coping mechanisms is fundamental to understanding and managing anger. Healthy coping strategies may include deep breathing exercises, physical activity, mindfulness, or seeking support from friends, family, or professionals. The key is to find methods that align with one's personality and lifestyle, providing a constructive outlet for managing and diffusing anger.

In conclusion, understanding anger is a multifaceted journey that involves exploring its psychological, physiological, and evolutionary aspects. It requires introspection, effective communication, cognitive restructuring, empathy, and the development of healthy coping mechanisms. By gaining insight into the roots of anger and adopting proactive strategies, individuals can transform their relationship with this powerful emotion, leading to personal growth, stronger relationships, and a more balanced emotional life.

CHAPTER 2
Recognizing Triggers

Recognizing triggers is crucial for maintaining emotional well-being. Triggers are stimuli or situations that evoke strong emotional reactions, often linked to past experiences. Identifying these triggers allows individuals to better understand and manage their responses, fostering healthier relationships and improved mental health.

Understanding triggers involves self-reflection and awareness. By pinpointing specific situations, words, or actions that cause emotional distress, individuals can develop strategies to navigate these challenges. It's essential to recognize that triggers vary from person to person, making self-awareness a personalized journey.

Common triggers include unresolved trauma, stress, or patterns learned in childhood. These triggers can manifest in various ways, such as anxiety, anger, or sadness. Recognizing them empowers individuals to break destructive cycles and cultivate positive coping mechanisms.

Journaling is a powerful tool for recognizing triggers. Recording thoughts and emotions during challenging moments provides insights into recurring patterns and their underlying causes. This written reflection aids in identifying triggers and developing proactive responses.

Communication plays a pivotal role in trigger recognition. Open and honest conversations with trusted individuals can shed light on blind spots and offer different perspectives. Seeking feedback helps build a support system that aids in identifying triggers and finding effective coping mechanisms.

Mindfulness practices, such as meditation and deep breathing, enhance self-awareness and assist in recognizing triggers in the present moment. Cultivating a mindful lifestyle allows individuals to respond thoughtfully rather than react impulsively to triggering situations.

Behavioral patterns can serve as clues to underlying triggers. Observing how one reacts in specific circumstances provides valuable information for trigger recognition. Consistent patterns may indicate unresolved issues that require attention and healing.

Recognizing triggers is an ongoing process. Life changes, and so do triggers. Regular self-check-ins and adjustments to coping strategies are essential for staying attuned to evolving triggers and maintaining emotional balance.

In summary, recognizing triggers is a fundamental aspect of emotional intelligence. Through self-reflection, open communication, mindfulness, and behavioral observation, individuals can identify and understand their triggers. This self-awareness forms the foundation for developing effective coping mechanisms, fostering emotional well-being, and building healthier relationships.

CHAPTER 3

Breathing Techniques

Breathing techniques play a crucial role in promoting physical and mental well-being. By adopting mindful breathing practices, individuals can enhance their overall health, manage stress, and improve focus. Let's explore some simple yet effective breathing exercises that can be easily incorporated into daily routines.

1. Diaphragmatic Breathing (Deep Belly Breathing):

One fundamental technique is diaphragmatic breathing. Start by sitting or lying down comfortably. Inhale slowly through your nose, allowing your abdomen to expand fully. Feel your diaphragm move downward, drawing air deep into your lungs. Exhale slowly through your mouth, ensuring a gentle and controlled release. This technique promotes relaxation and helps to reduce stress.

2. 4-7-8 Technique:

The 4-7-8 breathing technique, pioneered by Dr. Andrew Weil, is a simple method for calming the nervous system. Inhale quietly through your nose for a count of four, hold your breath for a count of seven, and then exhale audibly through your mouth for a count of eight. This rhythmic pattern helps regulate breathing, inducing a sense of tranquility.

3. Box Breathing (Square Breathing):

Box breathing is a versatile technique that can be practiced anywhere. Inhale for a count of four, hold your breath for four counts, exhale for four counts, and then maintain an empty breath for another four counts. Visualize drawing a square with each step of the breathing cycle. This method aids in reducing anxiety and enhancing focus.

4. Alternate Nostril Breathing (Nadi Shodhana):

This yogic breathing technique balances the left and right hemispheres of the brain. Sit comfortably and use your right thumb to close off your right nostril, inhaling deeply through your left nostril. Then, close your left nostril with your right ring finger and release the right nostril, exhaling completely. Continue this cycle for a few minutes, fostering mental clarity and a sense of calm.

5. Resonant Breathing (Coherent Breathing):

Resonant breathing involves maintaining a consistent breathing rate, typically around five breaths per minute. Breathe in and out slowly, aiming for a smooth and even rhythm. This technique synchronizes heart rate variability, promoting a state of coherence that can reduce stress and improve emotional well-being.

6. Mindful Breathing:

Mindful breathing involves paying close attention to each breath without trying to control it. Find a quiet space, sit comfortably, and focus your awareness on the sensations of breathing. Notice the rise and fall of your chest or the sensation of air passing through your nostrils. This practice fosters present-moment awareness and can be a powerful tool for managing stress.

7. Breath Counting:

An uncomplicated yet effective technique involves counting each breath. Inhale, then exhale, counting "one." Continue up to a count of ten, and then start again. If your mind wanders, gently bring your focus back to the count. This method enhances concentration and mindfulness.

8. Humming Breath (Bhramari Pranayama):

Bhramari pranayama involves producing a humming sound while exhaling. Close your eyes, take a deep breath in, and exhale with a humming sound like a bee. This practice has a calming effect on the nervous system and can be particularly beneficial for relieving tension and stress.

Incorporating these breathing techniques into your daily routine can contribute to a more relaxed and centered lifestyle. Whether you're facing a stressful moment, seeking improved focus, or aiming for better overall well-being, these simple practices offer valuable tools for enhancing the quality of your breath and, in turn, your life.

CHAPTER 4

Positive Communication

Positive communication is the art of conveying messages in an optimistic and constructive manner, fostering healthy relationships and creating a conducive environment. It involves expressing thoughts, feelings, and ideas in a way that promotes understanding, collaboration, and mutual respect.

Effective positive communication encompasses various aspects, starting with the choice of words. Using language that is encouraging and affirming can significantly impact the tone of a conversation. Words have the power to uplift and motivate, or conversely, to create tension and misunderstanding. Therefore, selecting words carefully and thoughtfully contributes to a positive communication style.

Non-verbal cues play a crucial role in positive communication. Maintaining eye contact, adopting an open posture, and using gestures that complement the message all contribute to conveying sincerity and receptiveness. A smile, for instance, can convey warmth and approachability, instantly creating a positive atmosphere.

Active listening is another cornerstone of positive communication. Being fully present in a conversation, giving undivided attention, and responding appropriately demonstrate respect and validation for the speaker. Reflective listening, where one paraphrases or summarizes the speaker's message, not only ensures understanding but also reinforces the value of the speaker's perspective.

Empathy is a powerful element in positive communication. Understanding and acknowledging others' emotions contribute to a supportive and compassionate dialogue. Expressing empathy involves recognizing and validating feelings, creating a connection that fosters trust and understanding.

In the workplace, positive communication is vital for effective teamwork. Clearly conveying expectations, providing constructive feedback, and recognizing achievements contribute to a positive work environment. This, in turn, enhances collaboration, boosts morale, and improves overall productivity.

Conflict resolution is another area where positive communication plays a pivotal role. Approaching conflicts with a positive mindset, focusing on solutions rather than blame, and using "I" statements instead of accusatory language can facilitate a more amicable resolution. This approach helps in maintaining relationships while addressing underlying issues.

In personal relationships, positive communication is the key to building strong connections. Expressing gratitude, offering compliments, and sharing positive experiences create an environment of appreciation and affection. It fosters a sense of security and mutual support, strengthening the bond between individuals.

Educational settings also benefit from positive communication. Teachers who use encouraging language, provide constructive feedback, and create an inclusive learning environment contribute to students' overall well-being and academic success. Positive communication in education goes beyond words; it involves creating an atmosphere where students feel valued, motivated, and empowered to learn.

Parenting is another context where positive communication is paramount. Setting clear expectations, using positive reinforcement, and maintaining open lines of communication with children foster a healthy parent-child relationship. Positive communication in parenting involves both verbal and non-verbal aspects, creating a nurturing environment for a child's emotional and social development.

In summary, positive communication is a versatile and essential skill applicable in various aspects of life. Whether in the workplace, personal relationships, education, or parenting, fostering a positive communication style contributes to healthier interactions, stronger connections, and overall well-being. It involves using affirming language, leveraging non-verbal cues, practicing active listening, and embracing empathy. By incorporating positive communication into our daily interactions, we can create a more harmonious and supportive world.

CHAPTER 5

Setting Boundaries

Setting boundaries is crucial for maintaining healthy relationships and personal well-being. Boundaries define the limits of acceptable behavior and help establish a sense of respect and autonomy. Whether in friendships, family dynamics, or work environments, clear and well-communicated boundaries contribute to positive interactions.

Personal boundaries are like invisible lines that separate your thoughts, feelings, and needs from those of others. They serve as a protective mechanism, preventing you from being overwhelmed or taken advantage of. Understanding and asserting your boundaries is a key aspect of self-care. Without clear boundaries, it's easy to feel emotionally drained or experience burnout.

In friendships, setting boundaries involves communicating your needs and expectations. This can include expressing your limits on time commitments, personal space, and emotional availability. Healthy friendships thrive when both parties understand and respect each other's boundaries. For instance, if you need alone time, it's important to communicate that without feeling guilty.

In familial relationships, boundaries help maintain a balance between independence and closeness. Clearly communicating your limits with family members can lead to more harmonious interactions. This might involve discussing topics that are off-limits, setting expectations for personal space, or establishing rules for communication.

At the workplace, setting boundaries is crucial for maintaining a healthy work-life balance. Clearly defining your work hours, expressing your limits on additional tasks, and communicating when you need support are all essential aspects of professional boundaries. Without these, burnout and stress can easily take a toll on your well-being.

One common challenge in setting boundaries is the fear of disappointing others. People often hesitate to assert their limits because they worry about being perceived as selfish or uncooperative. However, it's important to recognize that setting boundaries is not about being selfish but about maintaining a healthy balance that allows you to give and receive in a sustainable way.

Learning to say "no" is a powerful aspect of setting boundaries. Saying no doesn't mean you are rejecting someone; it simply means you are honoring your limits and prioritizing your well-being. It's a skill that requires practice, but it empowers you to make choices aligned with your values and priorities.

Effective communication is at the core of setting boundaries. Clearly expressing your needs, feelings, and expectations helps others understand where you stand. It also fosters an environment where open communication is valued, leading to stronger and more respectful relationships.

In addition to verbal communication, non-verbal cues also play a significant role in setting boundaries. Body language, facial expressions, and other non-verbal signals can convey your comfort level or discomfort with a situation. Being aware of these cues and respecting them in others enhances the overall understanding of boundaries.

Reassessing and adjusting boundaries is a normal part of personal growth and changing circumstances. As life evolves, so do our needs and limits. Regularly reflecting on your boundaries and making adjustments when necessary ensures that they remain relevant and effective.

Respecting the boundaries of others is equally important. Just as you have the right to set limits, you must also honor the boundaries established by those around you. This reciprocal respect creates a supportive and understanding environment where everyone feels valued.

In conclusion, setting boundaries is an essential aspect of maintaining healthy relationships and personal well-being. It involves clear communication, the ability to say no, and respecting both your own limits and those of others. By actively practicing boundary-setting skills, you empower yourself to create a balanced and fulfilling life.

CHAPTER 6
Time-Out Strategies

Time-out strategies are effective tools for managing behavior, offering individuals a chance to pause and reflect. In essence, time-out involves temporarily removing oneself from a situation or activity. This can be applied in various contexts, such as parenting, education, and workplace settings. The simplicity of this technique belies its profound impact on behavior modification.

In parenting, time-out serves as a constructive disciplinary measure. When a child exhibits challenging behavior, placing them in a designated time-out area for a brief period allows them to cool off and reconsider their actions. This method encourages self-regulation, teaching children to associate negative behavior with a pause in enjoyable activities.

Educationally, time-out strategies are employed to address disruptive behavior in classrooms. Students who exhibit disruptive conduct may be temporarily removed from the learning environment, providing them with an opportunity to reflect on their actions. This interruption fosters accountability and reinforces the importance of respectful behavior within a scholastic setting.

In the workplace, time-out strategies can be adapted to manage stress and conflicts. When tensions run high or disagreements arise, taking a short break to step back from the situation allows individuals to collect their thoughts and approach the issue with a calmer mindset. This practice promotes a healthier work environment and encourages effective communication.

The success of time-out strategies lies in their simplicity and universal applicability. By providing individuals with a moment to pause, reflect, and recalibrate, these strategies empower them to make more informed and constructive choices in various aspects of life.

CHAPTER 7

Stress Reduction

Stress reduction means finding ways to relax and calm your mind, like deep breathing, exercise, or spending time doing things you enjoy.

1. Deep Breathing:

Take slow, deep breaths to calm your nervous system and reduce stress.

2. Exercise Regularly:

Physical activity releases endorphins, helping to alleviate stress and improve mood.

3. Mindfulness Meditation:

Practice mindfulness to stay present and manage stress by focusing on the current moment.

4. Adequate Sleep:

Ensure you get enough quality sleep to rejuvenate your body and mind.

5. Healthy Eating:

Maintain a balanced diet rich in fruits, vegetables, and whole grains for optimal physical and mental health.

6. Time Management:

Organize tasks, prioritize, and break them into smaller, manageable steps to reduce overwhelm.

7. Social Connections:

Build and nurture supportive relationships; socializing can provide a valuable emotional outlet.

8. Limit Caffeine and Sugar Intake:

Reduce consumption of stimulants to prevent heightened anxiety.

9. Set Realistic Goals:

Establish achievable objectives to avoid setting yourself up for unnecessary stress.

10. Learn to Say No:

Don't overcommit; be assertive in setting boundaries and saying no when needed.

11. Laugh Often:

Humor can be a powerful stress-reliever, so indulge in activities that make you laugh.

12. Disconnect from Technology:

Take breaks from screens to reduce digital stress and promote real-world connections.

13. Practice Gratitude:

Reflect on positive aspects of your life to shift focus away from stressors.

14. Progressive Muscle Relaxation:

Tense and then release different muscle groups to promote physical and mental relaxation.

15. Engage in Hobbies:

Find activities you enjoy to unwind and divert your mind from stressors.

16. Seek Professional Help:

If stress becomes overwhelming, consider therapy or counseling for additional support.

17. Nature Walks:

Spend time outdoors, as nature has a calming effect on the mind.

18. Visualization Techniques:

Imagine a peaceful place or scenario to mentally escape stress.

19. Journaling:

Write down your thoughts and feelings as a way of processing and understanding them.

20. Prioritize Self-Care:

Allocate time for activities that bring you joy and relaxation, promoting overall well-being.

Incorporating these practical tips into your daily routine can contribute significantly to stress reduction and improved mental health. Remember that finding what works best for you may require some experimentation, so be patient and prioritize self-care consistently.

CHAPTER 8

Modeling Healthy Behavior

Modeling healthy behavior is crucial for fostering positive habits and well-being. When individuals exhibit and promote healthy choices, they serve as powerful examples for others. This positive influence can extend to various aspects of life, including physical activity, nutrition, mental well-being, and social interactions.

Firstly, engaging in regular physical activity sets the foundation for a healthy lifestyle. Modeling this behavior involves incorporating exercise into daily routines, whether it's walking, jogging, or participating in sports. By doing so, individuals not only improve their own fitness but also inspire those around them to prioritize movement. This can be particularly impactful in encouraging friends, family, and colleagues to adopt healthier habits.

In terms of nutrition, modeling healthy eating habits is equally essential. Choosing a balanced diet rich in fruits, vegetables, lean proteins, and whole grains sends a positive message about the importance of nourishing the body. Sharing meal plans, cooking tips, and recipes can further inspire others to make healthier food choices, fostering a collective commitment to well-rounded nutrition.

Mental well-being is another crucial aspect of a healthy lifestyle. Demonstrating stress management techniques, mindfulness practices, and the importance of self-care can positively impact those observing these behaviors. Modeling a healthy approach to handling challenges and maintaining emotional balance contributes to a supportive environment that encourages others to prioritize mental health.

Social interactions play a significant role in overall well-being. By modeling positive communication, empathy, and conflict resolution, individuals contribute to a healthier social environment. Building strong, supportive relationships fosters a sense of belonging and reduces stress, benefiting both individuals and the community at large.

In simpler terms, modeling healthy behavior is about leading by example. It's walking the talk when it comes to exercise, making mindful food choices, taking care of mental health, and cultivating positive social interactions. Through these everyday actions, individuals create a ripple effect, inspiring those around them to embrace healthier habits.

In conclusion, modeling healthy behavior is a powerful catalyst for positive change. Whether it's through physical activity, nutrition, mental well-being, or social interactions, individuals can make a lasting impact by showcasing the importance of healthy choices. By embodying these habits, individuals not only improve their own lives but also inspire and uplift others, creating a community committed to well-being.

CHAPTER 9

Seeking Support

Seeking support is a fundamental aspect of human experience. Whether facing personal challenges, professional dilemmas, or emotional struggles, reaching out for help can be a crucial step towards resolution and growth. The act of seeking support involves acknowledging vulnerability, embracing humility, and recognizing the value of connection in navigating life's complexities.

At its core, seeking support is about acknowledging that no one is an island. Humans are inherently social beings, and the strength of our interconnectedness lies in our ability to lean on one another in times of need. It is a testament to resilience and self-awareness when individuals recognize that they don't have to face their problems alone.

One of the primary reasons people seek support is to gain perspective. When faced with challenges, our vision can become narrow, and solutions may seem elusive. Seeking support opens the door to fresh insights, alternative viewpoints, and a broader understanding of the situation. Whether confiding in a friend, family member, or professional, the act of verbalizing concerns can illuminate hidden aspects of a problem and pave the way for innovative solutions.

Moreover, seeking support is an act of self-care. It involves prioritizing mental and emotional well-being, acknowledging one's limitations, and recognizing the importance of maintaining a healthy balance. Just as we seek medical advice for physical ailments, reaching out for support nurtures our mental and emotional health. This proactive approach to self-care fosters resilience and equips individuals with the tools needed to navigate life's inevitable challenges.

In the professional realm, seeking support is a sign of strength rather than weakness. Collaborative environments thrive on open communication, and individuals who are willing to seek guidance contribute to a culture of continuous improvement. It is through constructive feedback and mentorship that professionals can refine their skills, overcome obstacles, and achieve their goals. In this context, seeking support becomes a strategic move towards personal and collective success.

However, the act of seeking support is not without its challenges. Societal stigma around vulnerability can discourage individuals from reaching out. The fear of judgment, perceived weakness, or the misconception that seeking help implies incompetence are common barriers. Overcoming these obstacles requires a cultural shift that recognizes vulnerability as a source of strength and views seeking support as a proactive step towards personal and collective growth.

Technology has played a transformative role in shaping how support is sought and delivered. Online platforms and virtual communities provide spaces for individuals to connect, share experiences, and seek advice anonymously. The accessibility of information and support through digital channels has democratized the process, breaking down geographical barriers and connecting people across the globe. The rise of telehealth and virtual counseling services further highlights the evolving landscape of seeking support in the digital age.

In conclusion, seeking support is an integral part of the human experience, encompassing personal, professional, and emotional dimensions. It is an act of courage, self-awareness, and resilience. Embracing vulnerability and recognizing the value of connection are foundational elements in navigating life's challenges. As society continues to evolve, breaking down stigma and embracing support as a proactive step towards growth will contribute to healthier, more connected communities.

CHAPTER 10

Celebrating Progress

Celebrating progress is a fundamental aspect of human nature, deeply rooted in our collective desire for growth and improvement. Whether on a personal, societal, or global level, acknowledging achievements fosters a positive mindset, motivates continued efforts, and strengthens the bonds that unite us.

At the individual level, celebrating personal progress is a vital component of self-motivation. Setting and achieving goals provides a sense of accomplishment and boosts self-esteem. This celebration need not be extravagant; even small victories contribute to a positive feedback loop that propels individuals forward. Whether it's learning a new skill, overcoming a fear, or making healthier lifestyle choices, taking a moment to recognize and celebrate progress reinforces the belief that effort leads to positive outcomes.

On a societal level, celebrating progress becomes a shared experience that unites communities and fosters a sense of collective achievement. Milestones in education, science, technology, and social justice are all reasons to come together and acknowledge how far we've come. These celebrations serve as reminders of our capacity for positive change, inspiring a shared vision for the future. In this context, commemorating historical achievements is not just about nostalgia but also a means of instilling pride and a sense of identity within communities.

In the realm of science and technology, breakthroughs and advancements are celebrated for their transformative impact on society. The discovery of new medicines, advancements in renewable energy, or innovations in communication technology are all milestones that warrant recognition. Celebrating these achievements not only honors the hard work and dedication of those involved but also encourages further exploration and discovery. Moreover, it helps bridge the gap between the scientific community and the general public, fostering a deeper appreciation for the role of science in our daily lives.

Progress in the arts and culture also deserves celebration, as it reflects the evolving tapestry of human expression. Whether it's a groundbreaking piece of literature, a revolutionary work of art, or a genre-defying musical composition, these cultural advancements contribute to the richness of our shared human experience. Celebrating such milestones not only recognizes the creative brilliance behind these achievements but also encourages a vibrant cultural dialogue that transcends borders and connects people across diverse backgrounds.

Economic progress is another critical facet of societal development. Celebrating economic achievements, such as reaching new levels of prosperity, reducing poverty rates, or fostering job creation, underscores the positive impact on people's lives. This celebration becomes particularly meaningful when it involves inclusive growth, where the benefits are distributed equitably, ensuring that a rising tide lifts all boats.

Global progress, whether in addressing climate change, promoting human rights, or achieving peace, demands collective celebration. These endeavors require collaboration on an international scale, and acknowledging milestones in these areas reinforces the importance of global cooperation. Celebrating progress on a global stage also serves as a reminder that, despite our differences, we share common challenges and aspirations that transcend borders.

In the workplace, celebrating progress is a powerful tool for fostering a positive and motivated team culture. Recognizing individual and collective achievements creates a sense of camaraderie and reinforces the idea that everyone's contributions are valued. This celebration doesn't have to be limited to major accomplishments; acknowledging daily wins and milestones, no matter how small, contributes to a positive work environment and enhances overall productivity.

However, celebrating progress should not be seen as a reason to become complacent. Instead, it should serve as a catalyst for continuous improvement. While reveling in achievements, it's crucial to reflect on the journey that led to success and identify areas for further growth. This reflective approach ensures that celebrations are not just about the destination but also about the ongoing pursuit of excellence.

In conclusion, celebrating progress is an intrinsic and essential aspect of the human experience. It permeates all facets of life, from personal achievements to societal advancements and global cooperation. By recognizing and commemorating progress, we not only honor the hard work and dedication that went into achieving goals but also inspire future endeavors. Progress, when celebrated, becomes a source of motivation, fostering a positive mindset that propels individuals, communities, and the world toward even greater heights.

CONCLUSION

In summary, effective anger management for parents is crucial for fostering a harmonious family life. By acknowledging and addressing their own emotions, parents can create a positive and supportive environment for their children. Cultivating patience, practicing open communication, and setting positive examples are key components of successful anger management. When parents prioritize these aspects, they not only enhance their own well-being but also contribute to the emotional health and resilience of their children. It's an ongoing journey, but the rewards of a peaceful and loving family dynamic make it well worth the effort.